To my beloved husband and children. I would not be the woman I am today without your love and support. You are my heart, my joy, my everything.

Your Herbal Garden - A Companion Coloring Book Vol I
Published by Herbal Hearts Press 2025

Copyright © 2025 Stephanie Harjo
All rights reserved. No part of this book may be reproduced, stored in a retrieval system, or transmitted in any form or by any means—electronic, mechanical, photocopying, recording, or otherwise—without the prior written permission of the author or publisher.

All Inquiries should be directed to
Contact@herbalheartspress.com

Disclaimer:
This book is intended for educational and informational purposes only. The content provided is based on traditional herbal knowledge and is not a substitute for professional medical advice, diagnosis, or treatment. Always consult a qualified healthcare provider before using any plant or herbal remedy, especially for children, pregnant individuals, or those with medical conditions. The author and publisher are not responsible for any adverse effects resulting from the use of information in this book.

ISBN 979-8-9927836-2-9 Paperback

Your Herbal Garden
A Companion Coloring Book Vol I

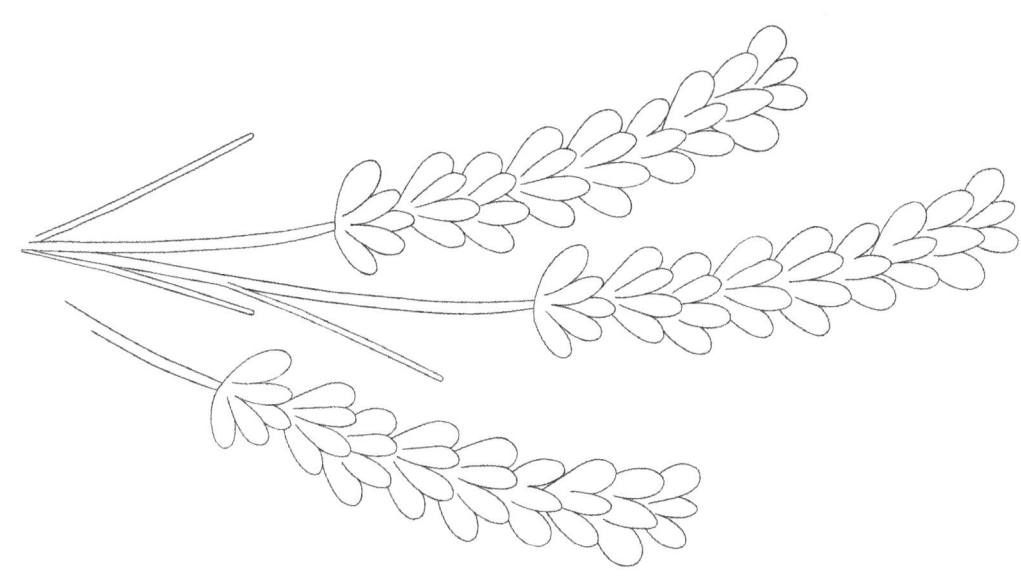

Written & Illustrated by
Stephanie Harjo

In your garden, colorful and bright
Grows a world of beauty and light.

Herbs with healing, you will see
Whispering secrets your body needs.

Let us explore, your garden awaits
For you to learn, grow, and create.

Lavender, with petals of purple
Is a sweet and calming herbal.

Her scent is earthy, sweet, and light
She calms your fears in the night.

Easing your mind, with her soft caress
She helps you get a good night's rest.

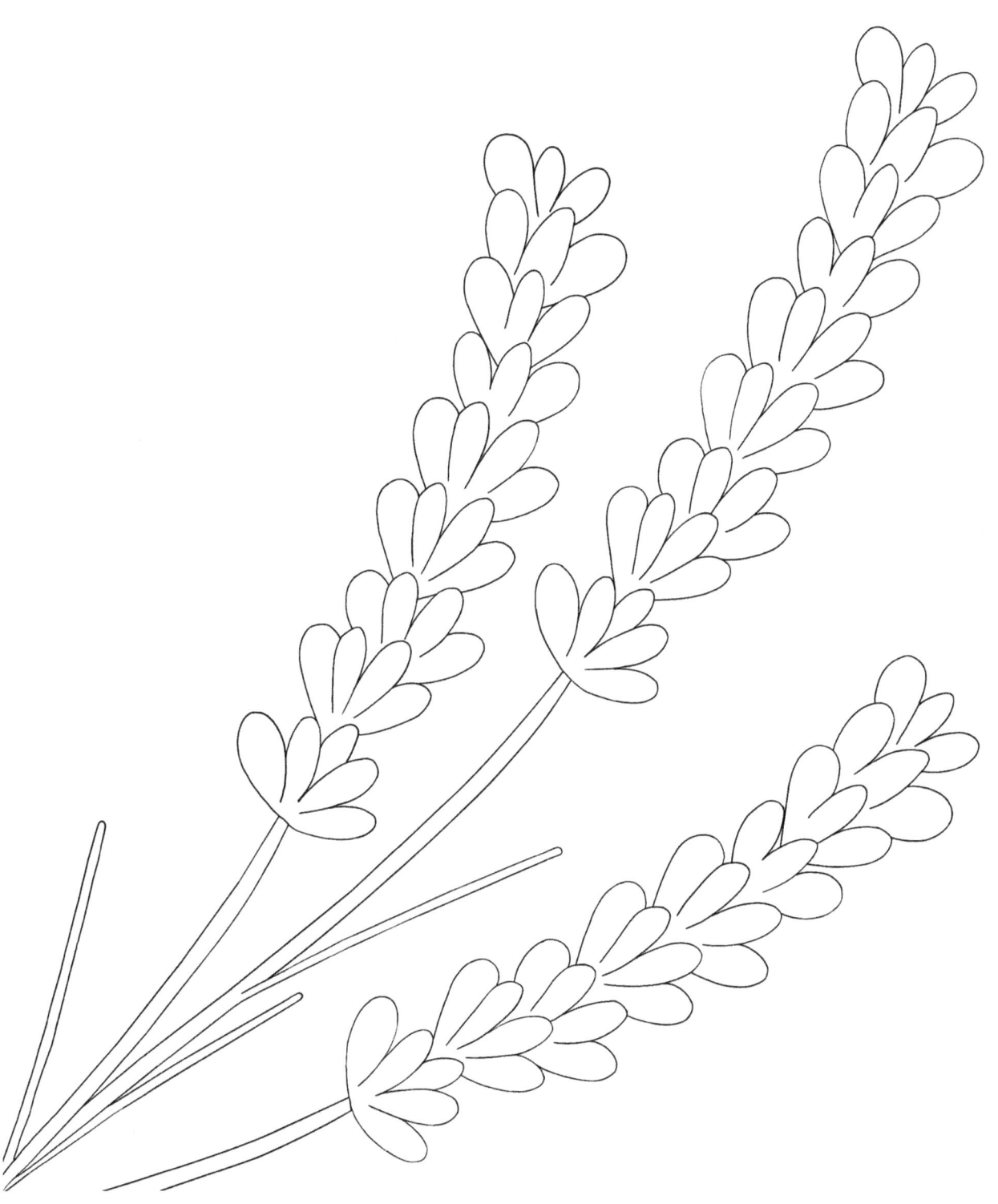

Rosemary, so earthy and bold
Is a beautiful herb to behold.

Her fragrance is strong, it fills the air
And clears your mind and lungs with care.

Inhale deep if your cough is strong
Your cold or flu will not stay long.

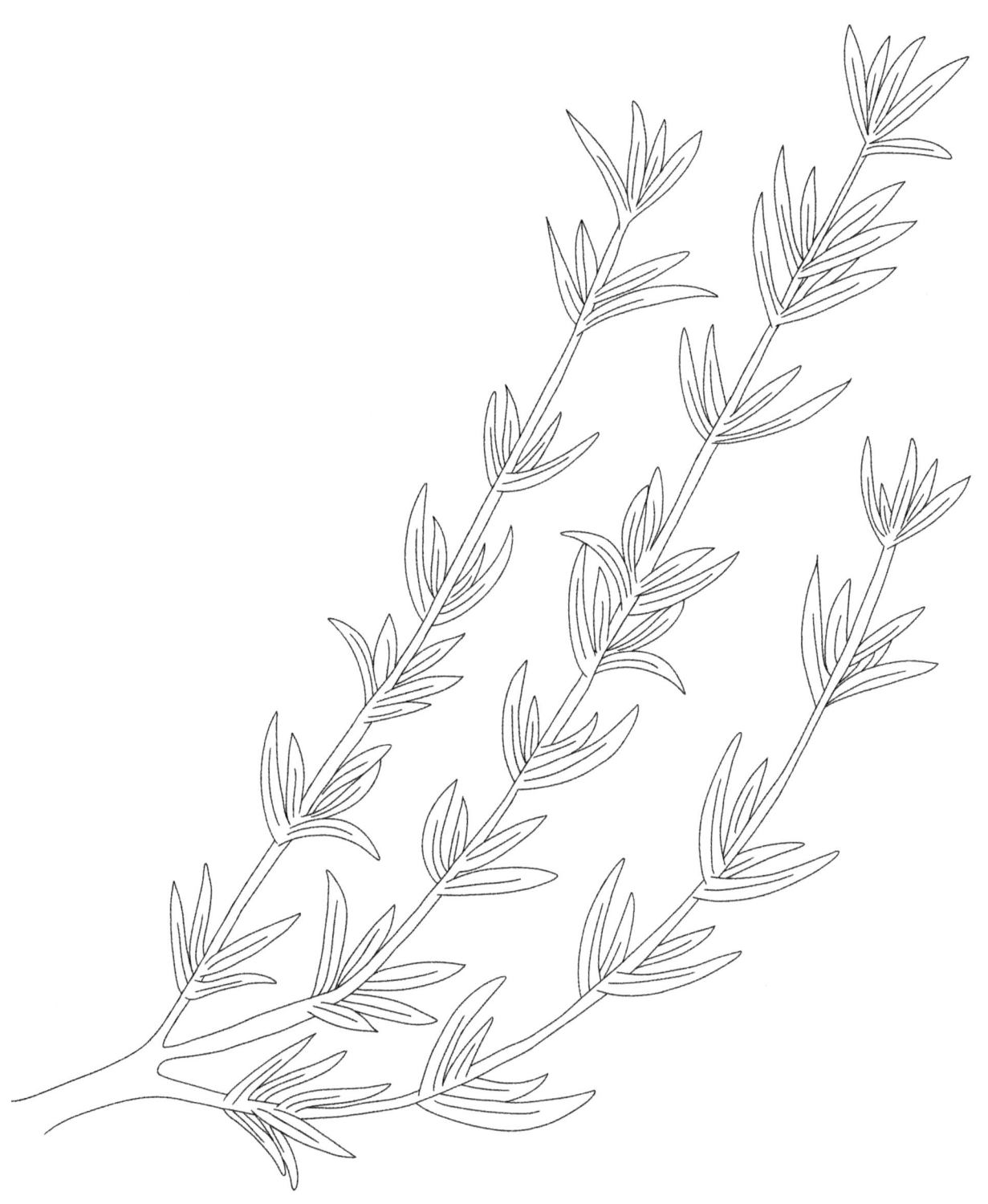

Chamomile, with blooms so small
Is a gentle medicine for one and all.

In your tea, she soothes and mends
Your best friend when a fever descends.

Golden petals, soft and sweet
Brings calm, peace, and a tender treat.

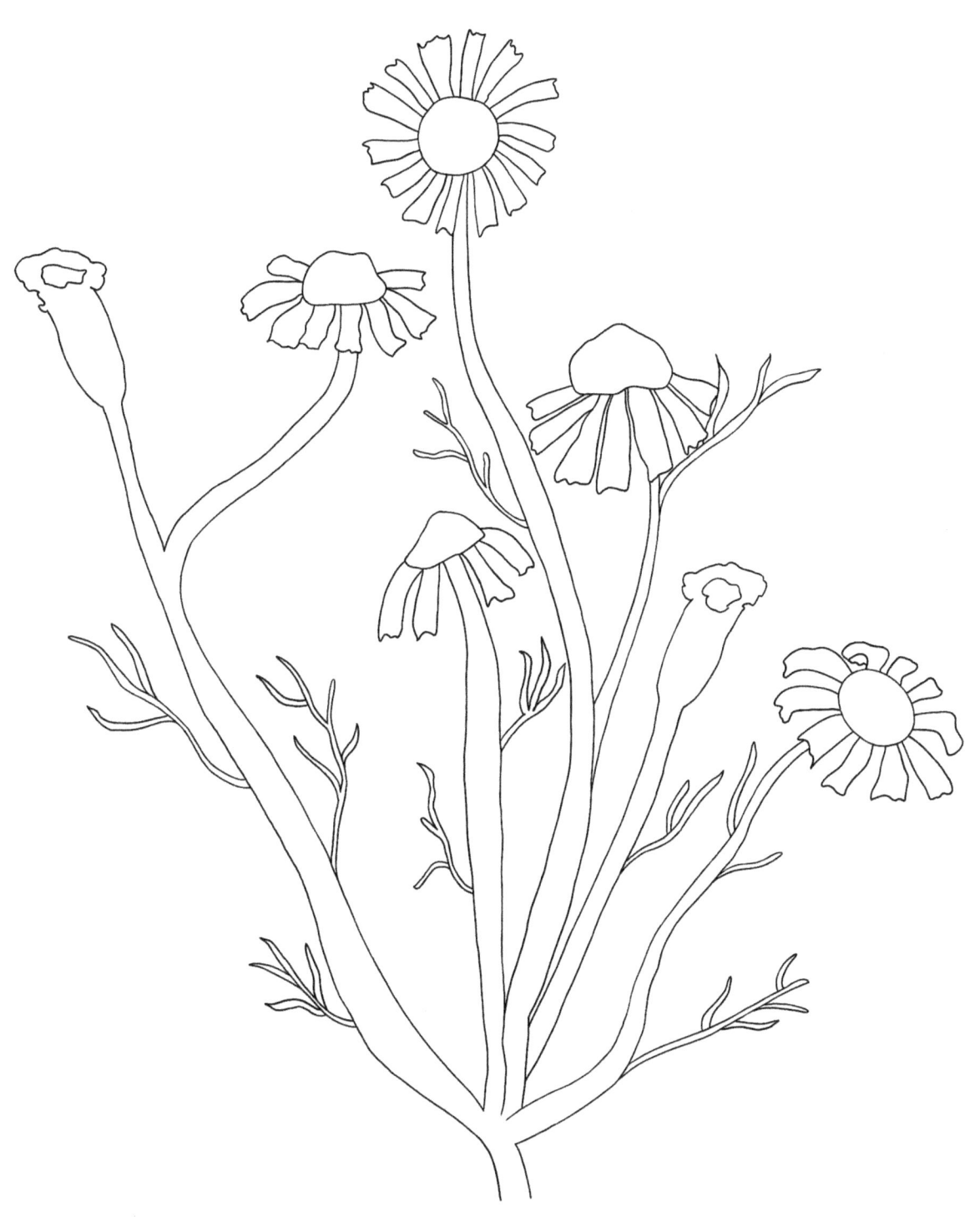

Peppermint, with leaves so green
His refreshing touch is crisp and clean.

In your tummy, his dance is light
Chasing away the aches at night.

Cool and bright, he lifts the soul
Peppermint makes the body whole.

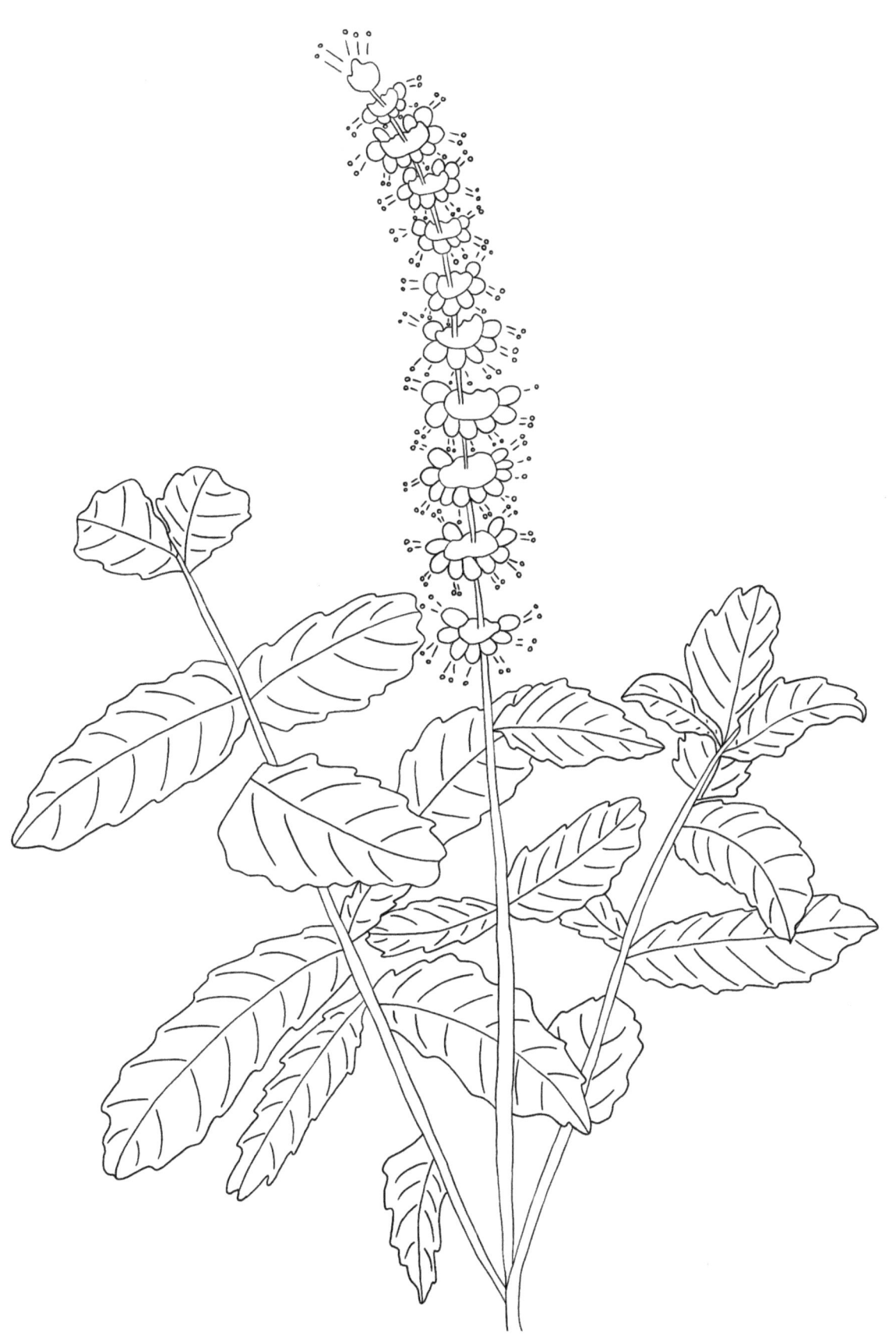

Echinacea, with a spiky looking crown
Has purple petals falling down.

A warrior plant, she fights off germs
Keeping your defenses nice and firm.

In a brew, her power flows
Drink it often and it will show.

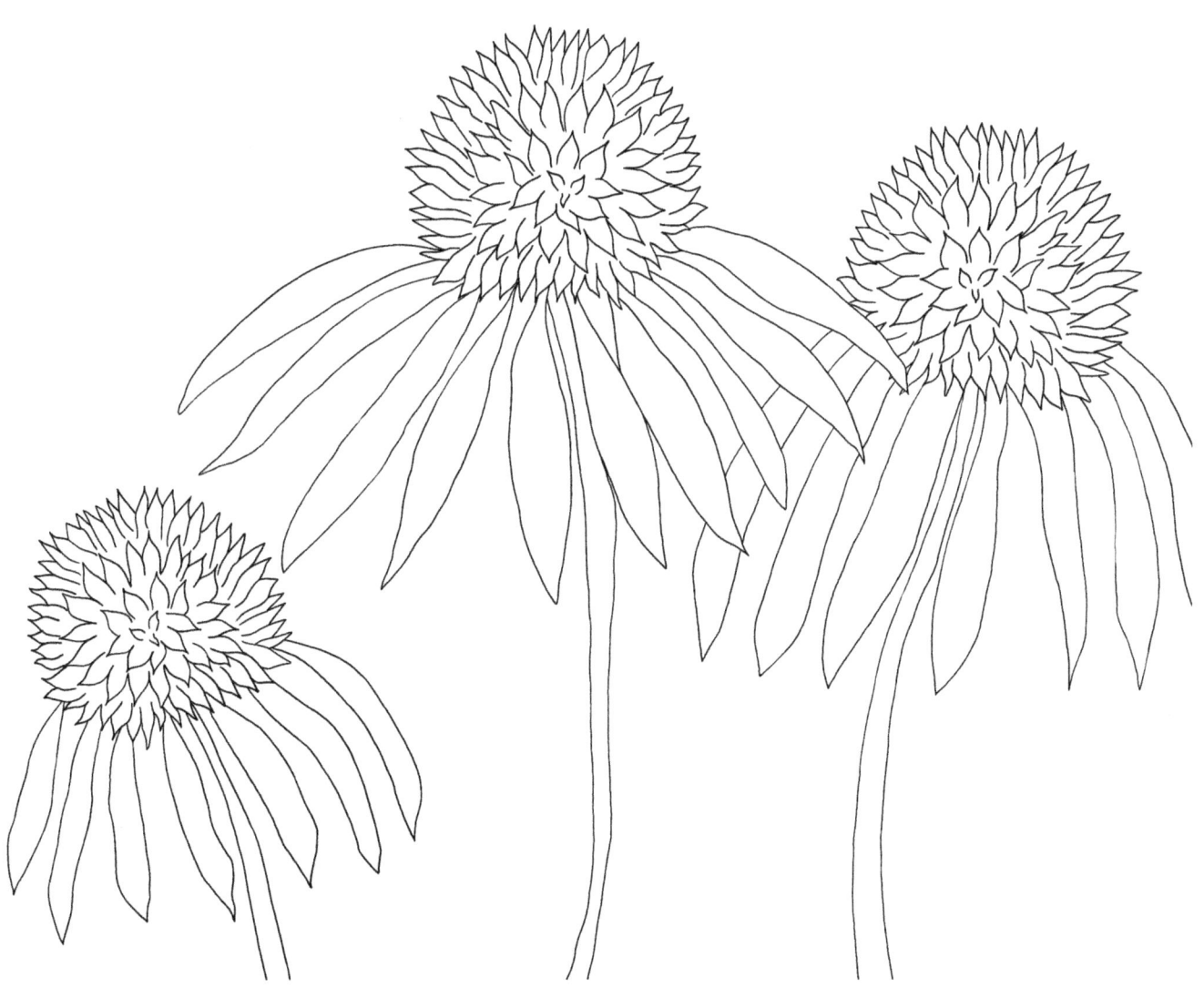

Calendula, so orange and bright
His medicine is full of might.

Add him to your salve, to soothe
He heals your broken skin and wounds.

But don't forget, drink your tea
He also heals wounds internally.

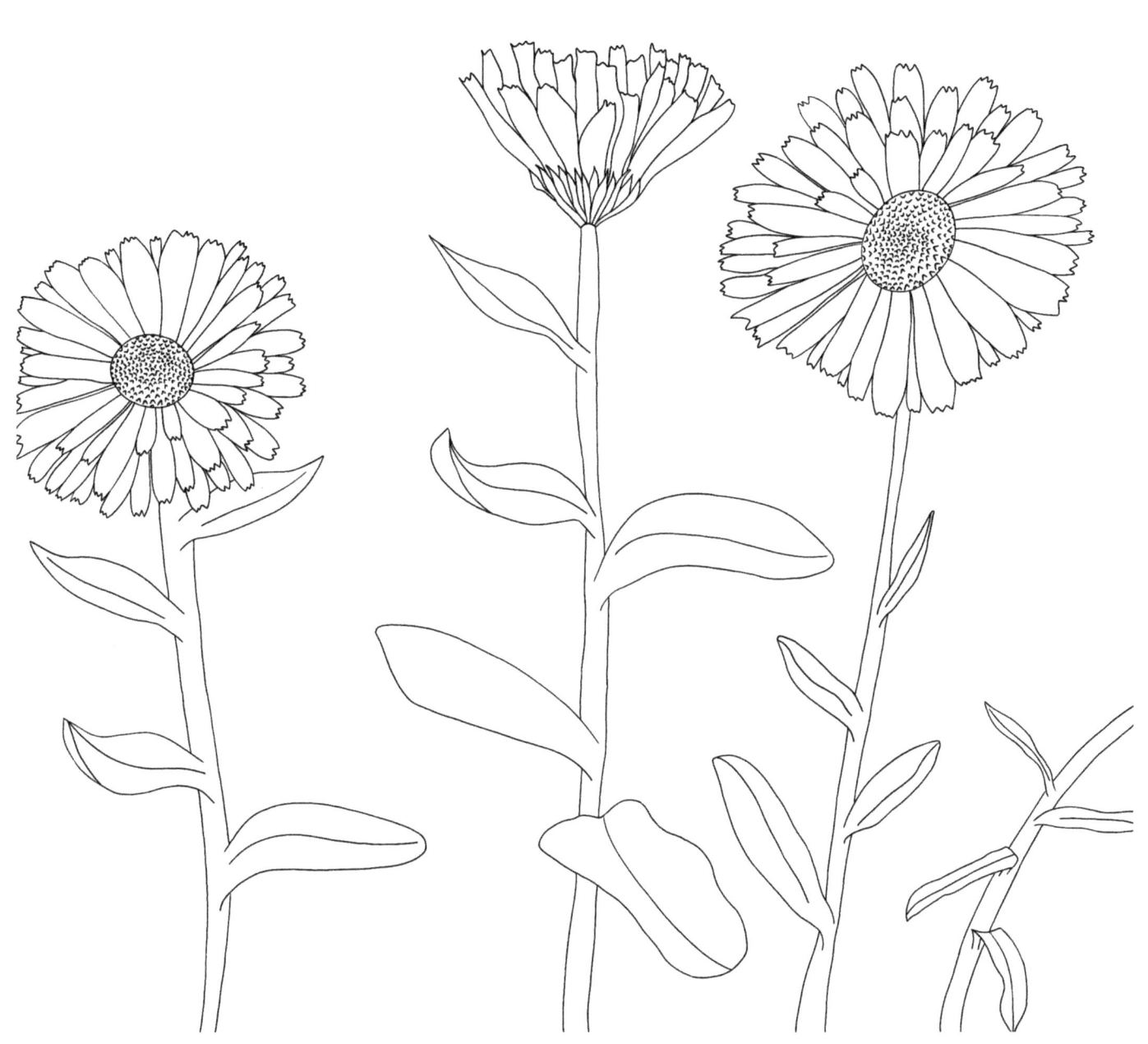

Ginger root, so fierce and soothing
He warms your blood and gets it moving.

A yucky tummy, with nausea or gas
Ginger root will soothe it fast.

Spicy warmth, a zesty zing
Ginger root is Ah-ma-zing!

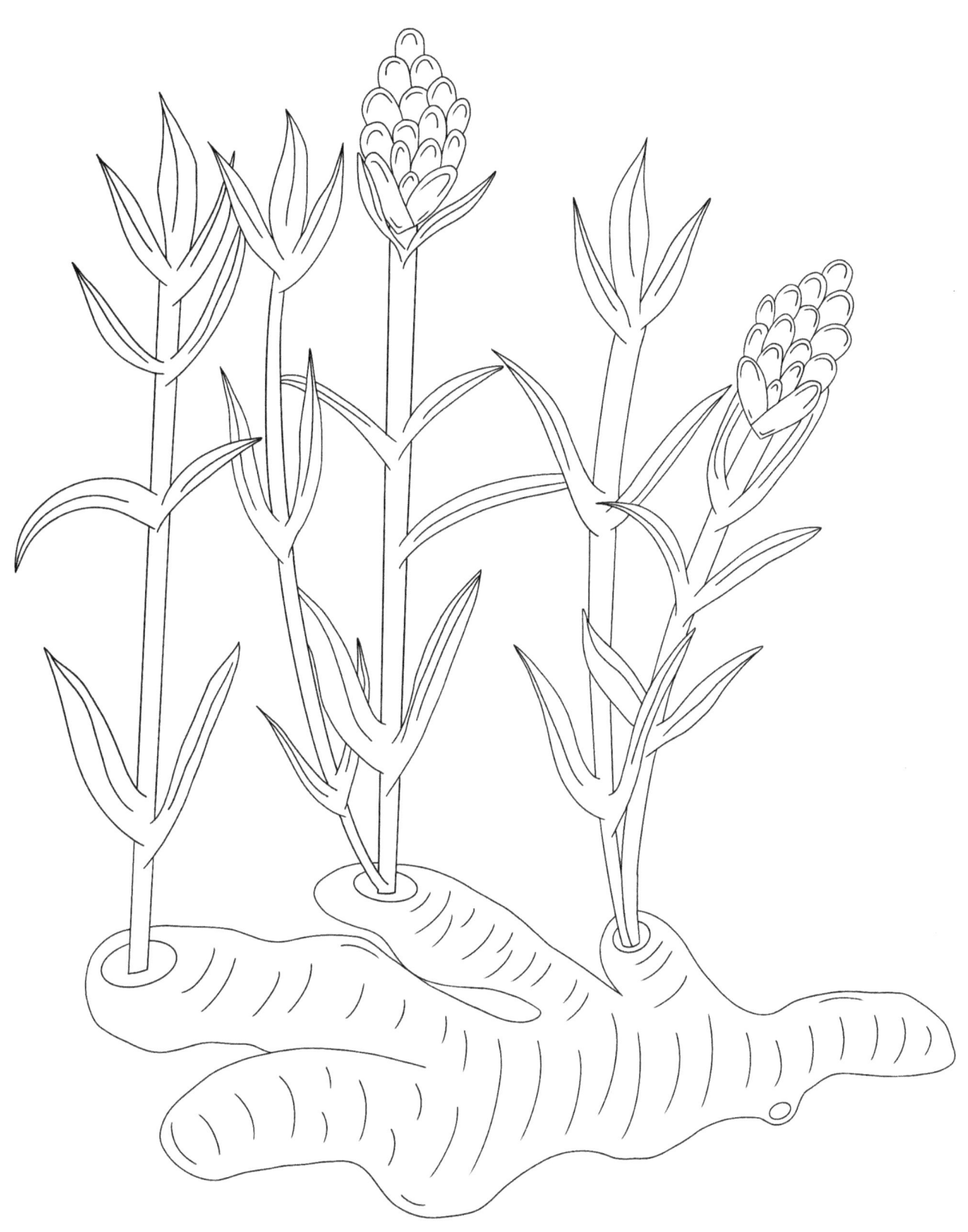

Elderberry, dark and sweet
Her many benefits are hard to beat.

In a syrup, tincture, or tea
Her medicine keeps you illness-free.

Berries are great, so are her flowers
Both are full of germ fighting powers.

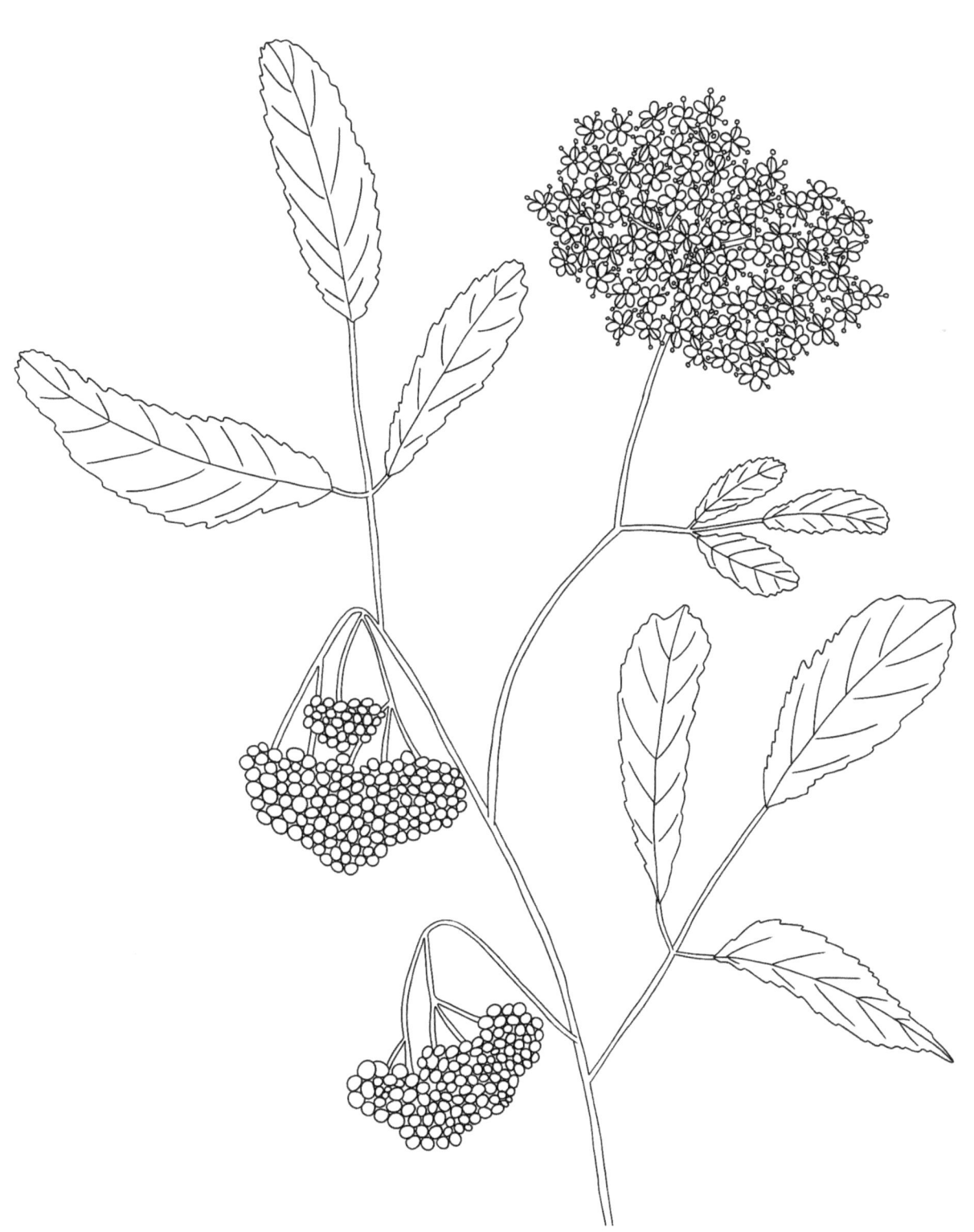

These herbs you explore, with loving care
Can be planted and grown anywhere.

Grow with love and they will flourish
Giving you medicine to heal and nourish.

With every smell, snip, and touch
Your herbal friends mean so much.

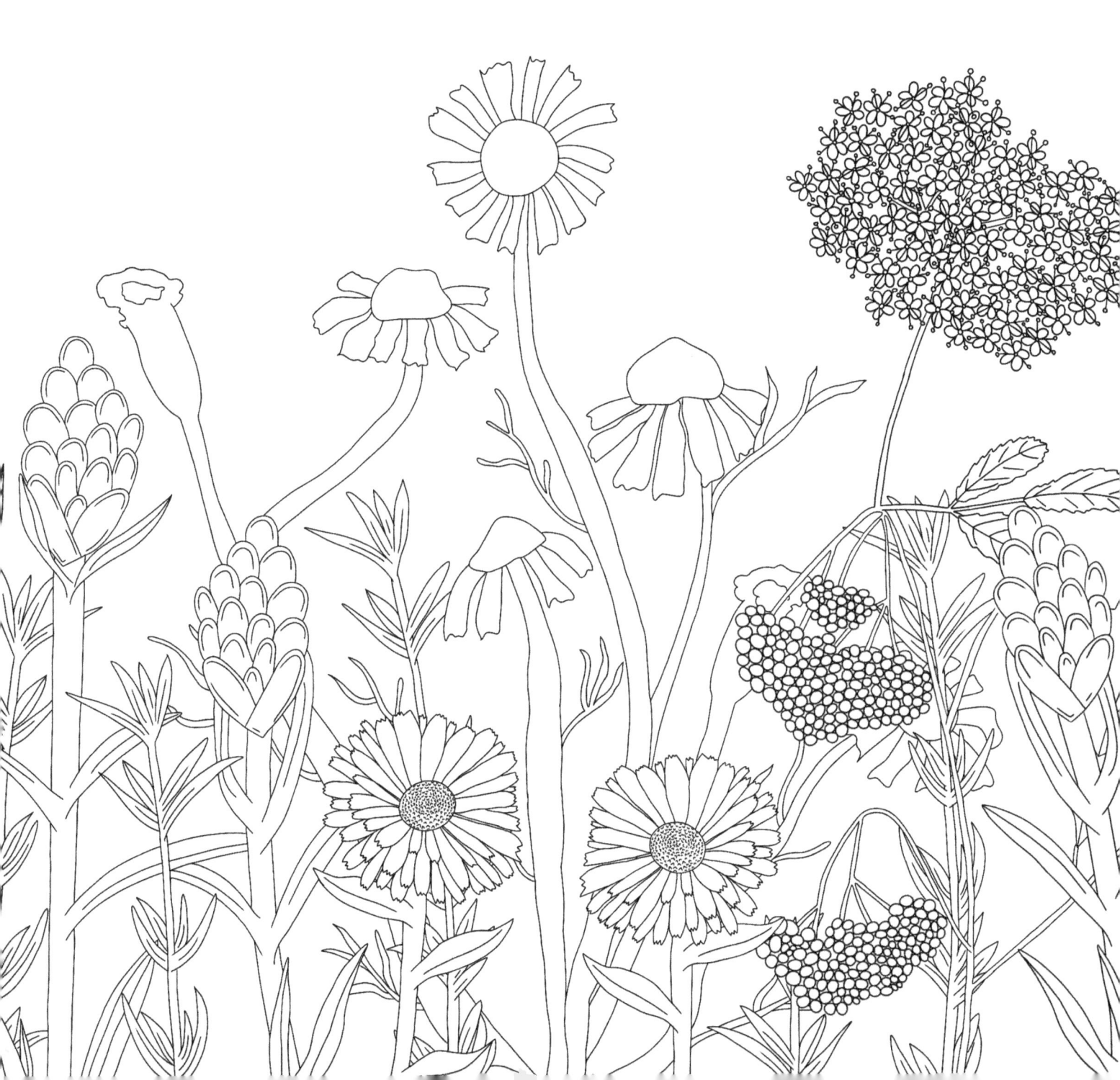

The end!

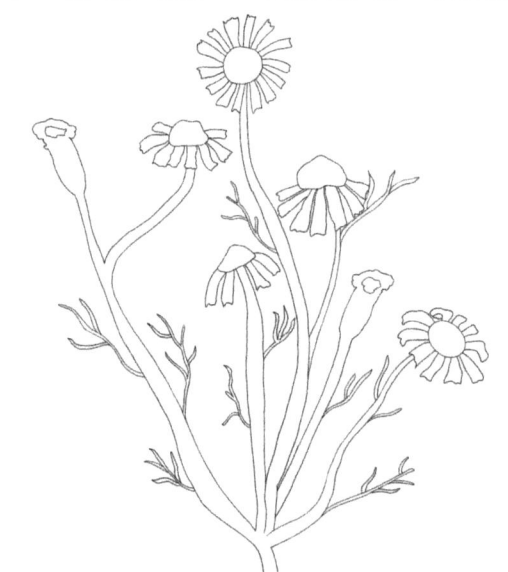

About the Author

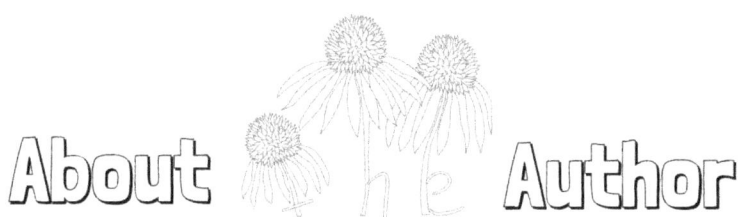

Stephanie lives on the Texas coast with her husband and two rambunctious teenagers. As a mother, she noticed a lack of children's books about herbs that could introduce young readers to the wonderful world of healing plants. Inspired by her love of herbal medicine, she set out to write a book that would spark curiosity and love for the natural world. When she's not writing, she enjoys spending time with her family, making herbal medicine, crafting, and getting lost in a good book.

For more about the author and her books visit Stephharjo.com

A Note from the Author:
Your voice matters! If you enjoyed this book, I'd be very grateful if you'd take a quick minute to leave a heartfelt review on Amazon. Your feedback and support mean the world to me and is incredibly important. Thank you for your time!

www.ingramcontent.com/pod-product-compliance
Lightning Source LLC
Chambersburg PA
CBHW040002040426
42337CB00032B/5198